GUT HEALTH COOKBOOK FOR WOMEN

A 2-Week Meal Plan and Gut-Friendly Recipes for Women to Improve Your Gut Microbes and Restore Your Digestive Balance and Wellness.

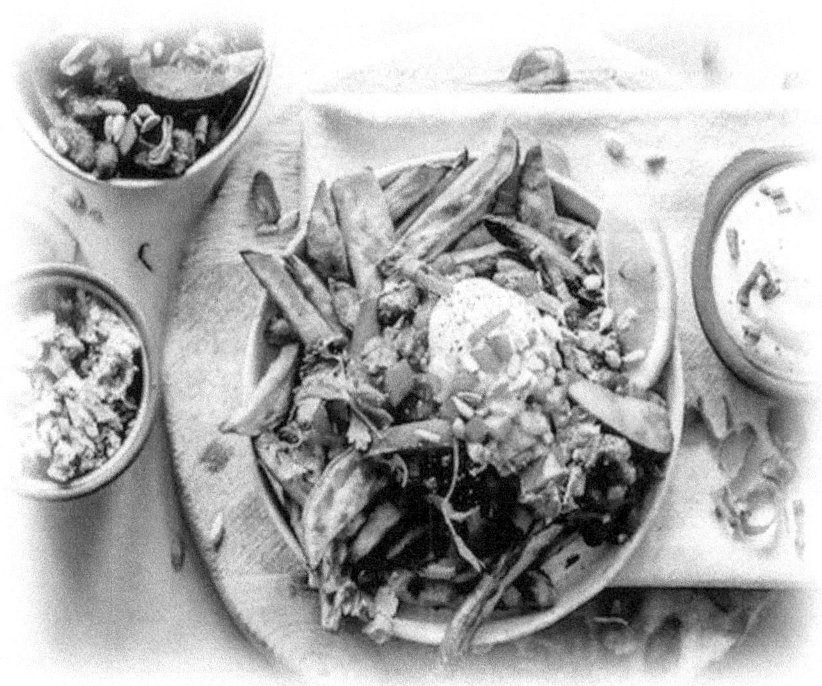

CHRISTIANA WHITE

GAIN ACCESS TO MORE BOOKS

TABLE OF CONTENTS.

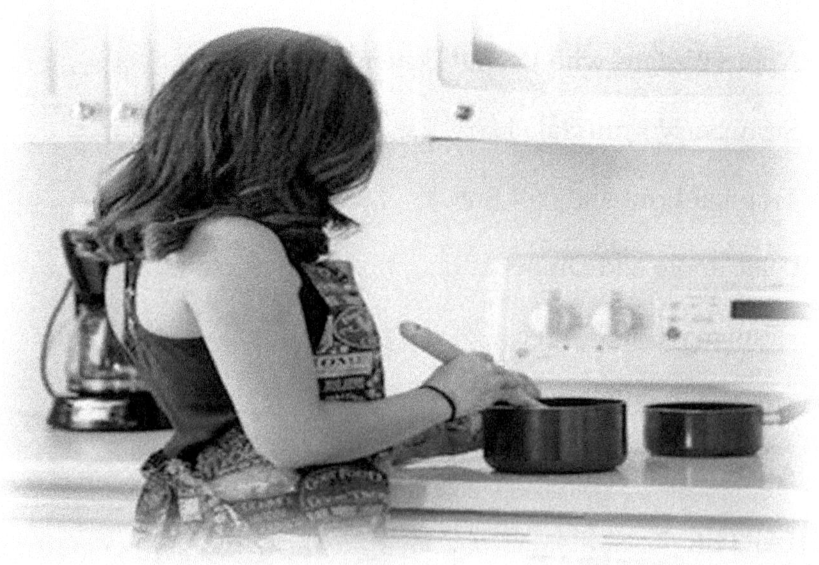

INTRODUCTION

Did you realize that your gut health influences more than just your digestion? It also affects your mood, immunity, metabolism, and possibly your risk of developing chronic diseases. In fact, the gut is sometimes referred to as your second brain due to the millions of nerve cells and microorganisms that communicate with your nervous system.

Welcome to the world of the Gut Health Diet Cookbook for Women, a life-changing resource that has helped countless women discover the secrets to a healthier, more harmonious connection with their bodies.

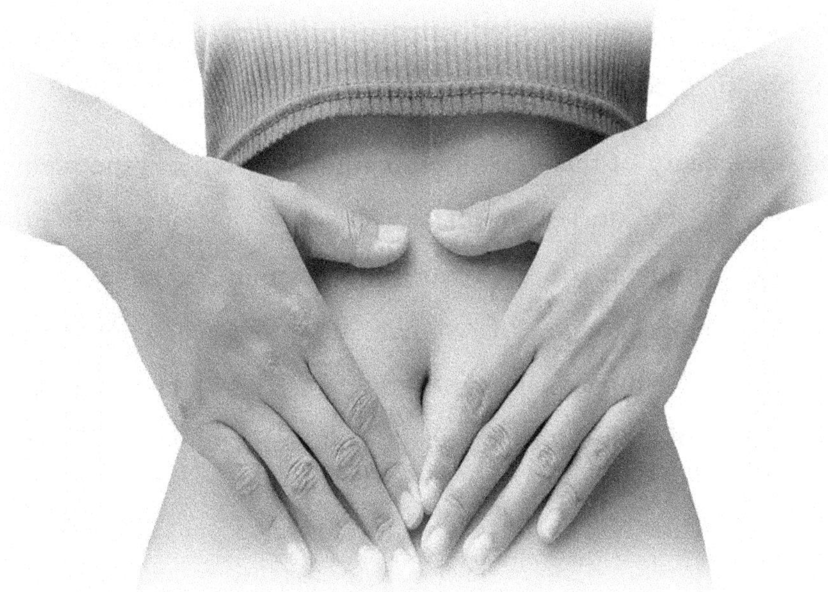

Hello, my name is Christiana White, and I am a trained nutritionist and gut health enthusiast. I wrote this book to share with you the journeys of many people who have healed their guts and transformed their health and wellbeing. This book is a gut health diet cookbook for women, with over 100 tasty and nutritious meals to nourish your gut and improve your overall health.

In the tapestry of stories created by this cookbook, women have discovered themselves not only cooking but also creating a symphony of Flavors that reverberate with vitality.

Sarah, a busy professional, found newfound energy and focus through the nutrient-dense dishes that became part of her daily routine. Emily, a woman negotiating the delicate balance of pregnancy, welcomed the individualized advice, loving the Flavors that benefited both her and her growing kid.

The true beauty of this cookbook is found not only in the recipes, but also in the stories of transformation it has inspired. From glowing comments of improved energy and digestive ease to heartbreaking accounts of women who overcame gut-related difficulties, the impact has been significant. This is more than just a compilation of recipes; it's a guide to comprehensive well-being.

If you want to take control of your gut health and your life, this book is for you. This book will teach you everything you need to know about gut health, including the science, benefits, and the finest foods and recipes. You'll also find tips and tactics to make your gut health journey more manageable and pleasurable.

You'll learn how to improve your digestion, increase your immunity, elevate your mood, and prevent or treat numerous chronic conditions. You will also learn how to design your own unique gut health plan based on your specific objectives, tastes, and needs. This book is more than simply a cookbook; it is a roadmap to becoming healthier and happier. So, what are you waiting for? Order your book today and start your gut health change!

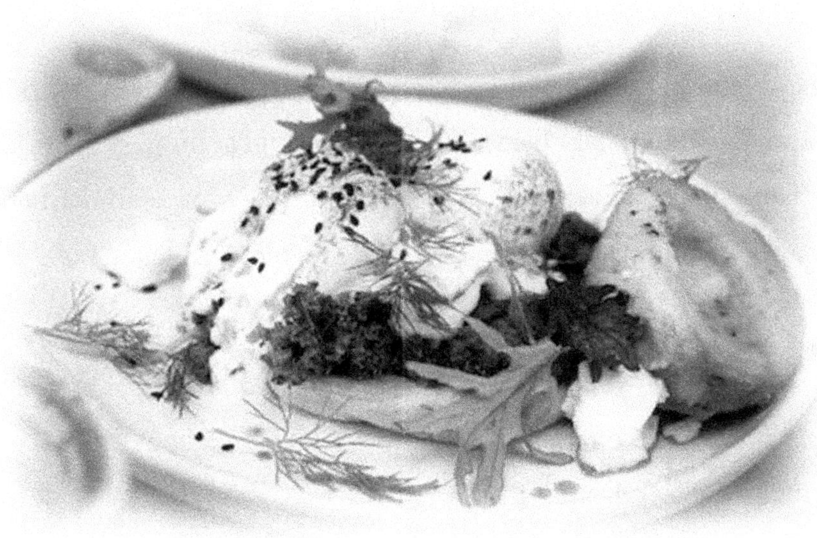

CHAPTER 1

The Significance of Gut Health for Women

Your gut is more than just a conduit for digesting and eliminating waste. It is also home to trillions of microbes known as the gut microbiome, which play an important role in your health and wellness.

These microbes help you digest food, generate vitamins, control hormones, reduce inflammation, and protect yourself from pathogens. They also communicate with your brain, immune system, and other organs via many paths.

Gut health is especially essential for women since it influences several areas of their health, including:

• **Hormonal balance:** Gut microorganisms can alter hormone production and metabolism, including oestrogen, progesterone, and cortisol. They can also influence how your body reacts to hormonal changes during the menstrual cycle, pregnancy, menopause, and stress.

An imbalance in your gut flora can be linked to hormonal problems such polycystic ovarian syndrome (PCOS), endometriosis, and premenstrual syndrome (PMS).

• **Mood and mental health**: The microorganisms in your gut can generate neurotransmitters like serotonin, dopamine, and gamma-aminobutyric acid (GABA), which influence your mood, emotions, and cognition.

They can also interact with your nervous system, influencing how you respond to stress, anxiety, and sadness. A dysbiosis in your gut microbiome can disrupt the brain-gut axis and raise your risk of mood disorders like IBS, CFS, and fibromyalgia.

• **Weight and metabolism**: Gut microorganisms can influence your appetite, satiety, energy expenditure, and fat accumulation. They may also affect your insulin sensitivity, glucose tolerance, and lipid profile. A change in your gut flora can affect metabolic functioning and increase your risk of obesity, diabetes, and cardiovascular disease.

• **Immunity and inflammation**: Gut microorganisms can help you fight infections, control your immune system, and protect your intestinal barrier. They can also influence your inflammatory response and prevent or worsen autoimmune disorders like rheumatoid arthritis, lupus, and multiple sclerosis. A disruption in your gut flora might weaken your immune system and cause chronic inflammation.

<u>*How a Healthy Gut Improves Overall Wellbeing*</u>

A healthy gut is one that has a diverse and balanced colony of microorganisms that serve a variety of positive functions for your body. A healthy stomach can improve your overall health in a variety of ways, including:

• **Improving digestion and nutrition absorption:** A healthy gut allows you to digest meals more efficiently and absorb nutrients more effectively. It can also help prevent or treat digestive issues like bloating, gas, constipation, diarrhoea, and stomach pain. A healthy gut can also help your liver function and detoxification processes.

• **Improving your mood and mental health:** A healthy gut produces and regulates neurotransmitters that influence your mood, emotions, and cognition. It can also help with stress management, anxiety, and depression. A healthy stomach can also help with cognitive skills like memory, learning, and attention.

• **Improving your weight and metabolism**: A healthy gut can help you control your appetite, satiety, energy expenditure, and fat storage levels. It can also help with insulin sensitivity, glucose tolerance, and lipid profile. A healthy gut can also help you avoid metabolic illnesses like obesity, diabetes, and cardiovascular disease.

• **Boosting immunity and inflammation:** A healthy gut can help you fight infections, control your immune system, and protect your intestinal barrier. It can also control your inflammatory response and help prevent or treat autoimmune illnesses.

A healthy gut may also reduce your chances of chronic diseases including cancer, asthma, and allergies.

As you can see, having a healthy gut can improve your overall health in a variety of ways. As a result, it is critical to follow a healthy gut diet that will fuel your gut flora while also increasing its diversity and balance.

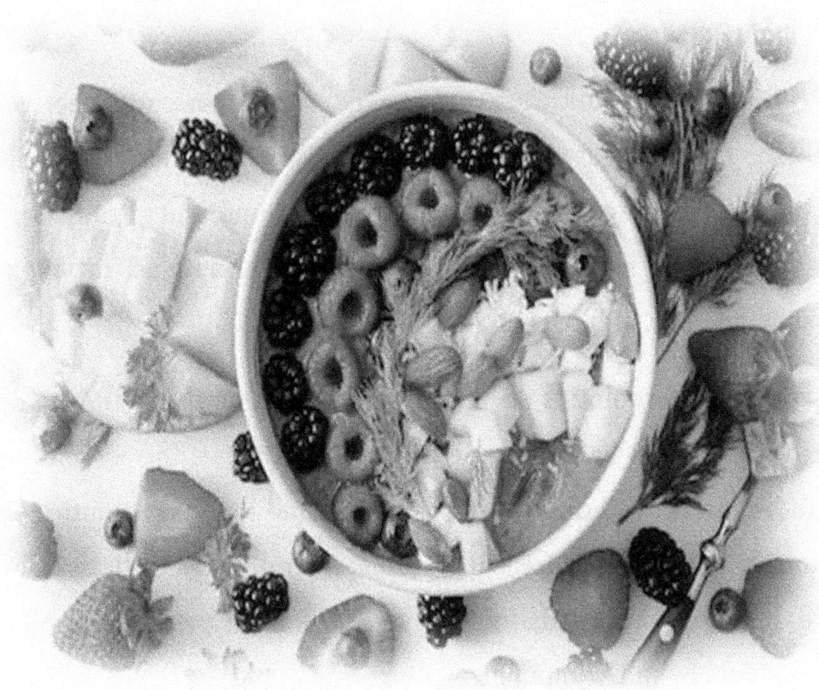

CHAPTER 2

Foundations of Nutrition

A healthy gut diet for women is built on dietary principles that promote the growth and function of your gut flora. The foundations are:

• **Fiber**: Fiber is an indigestible component of plant meals that can nourish your gut microorganisms and increase their diversity and activity. Fiber can also help you control your bowel motions, reduce your cholesterol, and manage your blood sugar. Fiber-rich foods include fruits and vegetables, whole grains, legumes, nuts, and seeds.

• **Prebiotics**: Prebiotics are specialized fibres that can selectively nourish healthy gut flora like bifidobacteria and lactobacilli. Prebiotics can also benefit your digestion, immunity, and mood. Prebiotic foods include garlic, onion, leek, asparagus, artichoke, banana, chicory, and oats.

• **Probiotics**: Probiotics are live microorganisms that replace your gut microbiome and provide a variety of health advantages, including improved digestion, immunity, and mood. Probiotics can also help you avoid or treat infections, allergies, and inflammatory illnesses. Probiotic foods include yogurt, kefir, sauerkraut, kimchi, miso, tempeh, and kombucha.

• **Polyphenols**: Polyphenols are naturally occurring chemicals in plant foods that contain antioxidant, anti-inflammatory, and antibacterial effects. Polyphenols can also alter your gut microbiota, affecting your metabolism, immunity, and mood. Polyphenol-rich foods include berries, grapes, apples, citrus fruits, green tea, chocolate, red wine, and spices.

• **Healthy Fats:** Healthy fats are required for proper cell membrane, hormone, and brain function. Healthy fats can also benefit your gut microbiota and lower inflammation. Healthy fats include omega-3 fatty acids, monounsaturated fats, and medium-chain triglycerides.

Omega-3-rich foods include fatty fish, flaxseeds, chia seeds, and walnuts. Monounsaturated foods include olive oil, avocado, and almonds. Coconut oil and palm oil are good sources of medium-chain triglycerides.

These nutritional foundations can help you create a healthy gut diet for women that will fuel your gut bacteria while also benefiting your overall health.

Key Nutrients for Gut Health

In addition to the dietary underpinnings, other vital nutrients can help with gut health and function. The nutrients are:

• **Vitamin A:** Vitamin A is beneficial to your vision, skin, and immune system. Vitamin A can also help you maintain an intestinal barrier and avoid leaky gut syndrome. Vitamin A-rich foods include liver, eggs, dairy products, carrots, sweet potatoes, and spinach.

• **Vitamin D**: Vitamin D is vital for bone health, calcium absorption, and immunological function. Vitamin D can also help you control your gut microbiota and decrease inflammation. Vitamin D-rich foods include fatty fish, egg yolks, mushrooms, and fortified products. Vitamin D can also be obtained by sunshine exposure.

• **Vitamin C:** Vitamin C is essential for collagen production, wound healing, and antioxidant defence. Vitamin C can also aid to maintain your gut microbiota and protect your intestinal lining. Citrus fruits, kiwis, strawberries, broccoli, and peppers are good sources of vitamin C.

• **Vitamin B12:** Vitamin B12 is essential for red blood cells, neuron function, and DNA synthesis. Vitamin B12 can also help you avoid anaemia, exhaustion, and neurological issues. Meat, poultry, fish, eggs, dairy products, and fortified meals are all good sources of vitamin B12. You may also require a supplement if you are vegan or vegetarian.

• **Zinc**: Zinc is necessary for proper growth, development, and wound healing. Zinc can also assist manage the gut microbiome and immune system. Zinc-rich foods include oysters, cattle, lamb, pumpkin seeds, and lentils.

• **Magnesium**: Magnesium is required for proper muscle and nerve function, energy production, and bone health. Magnesium can also benefit your digestion, bowel movements, and mood. Dark chocolate, almonds, cashews, spinach, and avocado are good sources of magnesium.

These essential nutrients can help you improve your gut's health and function. They can be obtained through a well-balanced and varied diet, or by taking supplements if necessary.

Gut-Friendly Foods for Women

Based on the nutritional foundations and essential nutrients, here are some gut-friendly foods for women that you can incorporate into your healthy gut diet:

• **Fruits**: Fruits contain fibre, prebiotics, polyphenols, vitamin C, and antioxidants. They can nourish your gut microbes, boost your immune system, and reduce inflammation. Berries, apples, bananas, oranges, and grapes are among the most beneficial fruits for your gut.

• **Vegetables** contain fibre, prebiotics, polyphenols, vitamin A, and antioxidants. They can nourish gut microbes, strengthen your intestinal barrier, and reduce inflammation. Leafy greens, cruciferous vegetables, carrots, sweet potatoes, and artichokes are among the most beneficial vegetables for your gut.

• **Whole grains** are rich in fibre, prebiotics, polyphenols, magnesium, and B vitamins. They can nourish your gut microbes, aid digestion, and regulate blood sugar. Oats, quinoa, buckwheat, and brown rice are some of the most beneficial whole grains for your gut.

• **Legumes:** Rich in fibre, prebiotics, protein, iron, and zinc. They can nourish your gut microbes, improve digestion, and prevent anaemia. Beans, lentils, chickpeas, and soybeans are among the most beneficial legumes for your gut.

• **Nuts and seeds** are high in fibre, good fats, protein, magnesium, and zinc. They can nourish your gut microbes, improve brain function, and reduce inflammation.

Nuts and seeds that are good for your gut include almonds, walnuts, flaxseeds, chia seeds, and pumpkin seeds.

• **Fermented foods** contain probiotics, prebiotics, polyphenols, and vitamin B12. They can replenish your gut microbiome, boost your immune system, and improve your mood. Yogurt, kefir, sauerkraut, kimchi, miso, and tempeh are among the most beneficial fermented foods for your gut.

• **Healthy oils** contain healthy fats, polyphenols, and vitamin E. They can help your gut microbiome, decrease inflammation, and protect your cells. Olive oil, coconut oil, and avocado oil are among the most beneficial healthy oils for your gut.

These are some examples of gut-friendly foods for women that you can include in your healthy gut diet.

You can also add some spices, herbs, and teas to enhance the flavour and the benefits of your food. You should also drink plenty of water to hydrate your body and your gut.

Chapter 3

Breakfast Recipes

Berry Chia Seed Overnight Oatmeal

- *Servings: Two.*
- *Prep time: 5 minutes, plus overnight.*

Ingredients:

- One cup rolled oats.
- Two teaspoons of chia seeds.
- Two cups of unsweetened almond milk.
- 1/4 teaspoon of vanilla extract.
- One-quarter teaspoon cinnamon
- Two teaspoons of maple syrup or honey.
- 1/2 cup fresh or frozen mixed berries.
- Two tablespoons of chopped almonds or walnuts.

Step-by-Step Instructions:

- In a large mixing bowl, combine the oatmeal, chia seeds, almond milk, vanilla, cinnamon, and maple syrup or honey.

- Divide the oat mixture into two lidded jars or containers. Top with fruit and nuts. Cover and refrigerate overnight, or at least 4 hours.
- Enjoy either cold or warm in the morning. If needed, add extra almond milk.

Scrambled Eggs with Spinach and Tomatoes.

- *Servings: Two.*
- *Prep time: 10 minutes.*

Ingredients:

- Four eggs, beaten
- Two teaspoons of milk or water.
- Add salt and pepper to taste.
- One tablespoon of butter or olive oil.
- Two cups baby spinach.
- 1/4 cup cherry tomatoes, halved
- Two tablespoons of grated cheese (optional)
- 2 pieces of whole wheat bread toasted (optional)

Step-by-Step Instructions:

- In a small bowl, whisk together the eggs, milk or water, salt, and pepper.

- In a large skillet over medium-high heat, melt the butter or oil. Cook until the spinach wilts and the tomatoes soften, about 5 minutes.

- Reduce the heat to low, then pour the egg mixture over the spinach and tomatoes. Scramble the eggs gently until cooked to your preference, which should take between 3 to 5 minutes. Sprinkle with cheese if desired.

- You can serve the scrambled eggs with bread or on their own.

Green Smoothie Bowl

- *Servings: Two.*
- *Prep time: 10 minutes.*

Ingredients:

- Two cups baby spinach.
- One large banana, peeled and frozen
- 1/2 cup of frozen pineapple pieces.
- 1/4 cup plain yogurt, or kefir
- 1/4 cup of unsweetened almond milk.
- Two teaspoons of hemp seeds or flaxseeds

- Your preferred toppings, including fresh berries, granola, coconut flakes, or nut butter.

Step-by-Step Instructions:

- In a blender, add spinach, banana, pineapple, yogurt or kefir, almond milk, and hemp or flaxseeds.
- Blend until smooth and creamy, adding additional almond milk as needed to suit consistency.
- Divide the smoothie into two bowls and top with your preferred toppings. Enjoy with a spoon.

Baked Sweet Potatoes with Nut Butter and Sliced Apples

- *Servings: Two.*
- *Prep time: 45 minutes*

Ingredients:

- Wash two medium sweet potatoes and puncture them with a fork.
- 2 tablespoons of your preferred nut butter, like almond, peanut, or cashew.
- one large apple, cored and sliced
- Two teaspoons of honey or maple syrup.
- One-quarter teaspoon cinnamon

Step-by-Step Instructions:

- Preheat the oven to 200°C (180°C fan) and prepare a baking sheet with parchment paper. Place the sweet potatoes on the prepared baking sheet and cook for 40 to 45 minutes, or until cooked.

- Cut the sweet potatoes in half, then scoop out some of the flesh to create room for the filling. Transfer the scooped flesh to a small bowl and mash it with a fork.

- In a small saucepan over low heat, add the nut butter, honey or maple syrup, and cinnamon and whisk until smooth and blended.

- Fill each sweet potato half with mashed sweet potatoes and drizzle with nut butter. Top with apple slices and serve.

Quinoa Porridge with Berries and Nuts.

- *Servings: Two.*
- *Prep time: 20 minutes.*

Ingredients:

- 1 cup washed and drained quinoa.
- Two glasses of water.
- 1/4 teaspoon of salt.

- 1/4 cup of unsweetened almond milk.

- Two teaspoons of maple syrup or honey.

- 1/4 teaspoon of vanilla extract.

- One-quarter teaspoon cinnamon

- 1/2 cup fresh or frozen mixed berries.

- Two tablespoons of chopped almonds or walnuts.

Step-by-Step Instructions:

- In a small saucepan, heat the quinoa, water, and salt until boiling. Reduce the heat to a simmer and cover for 15 to 20 minutes, or until the quinoa is cooked and the water has been absorbed.

- Fluff the quinoa with a fork, then add the almond milk, maple syrup or honey, vanilla, and cinnamon.

- Divide the quinoa porridge between two dishes, then top with berries and almonds. Enjoy either hot or cold.

Avocado Toast with Sprouts and Smoked Salmon.

- *Servings: Two.*
- *Prep time: 10 minutes.*

Ingredients:

- Two pieces of whole wheat bread, toasted
- One ripe avocado, peeled and pitted
- Add salt and pepper to taste.
- 1/4 cup microgreens or alfalfa sprouts.
- Two ounces of smoked salmon.
- Two teaspoons of lemon juice.
- Two teaspoons of capers (optional)

Step-by-Step Instructions:

- In a small mixing bowl, mash the avocado with a fork and season with salt and pepper.
- Spread the avocado equally on the bread pieces, then top with sprouts or microgreens and smoked salmon.
- Drizzle with lemon juice and garnish with capers if preferred. Enjoy with a fork and knife or by hand.

Yogurt Parfait with Granola and Fruit

- ***Servings: Two.***
- ***Prep time: 5 minutes.***

Ingredients:

- Two cups plain yogurt or kefir.
- 1/4 cup granola of your preference
- 1/4 cup fresh or frozen mixed berries.
- Two tablespoons of honey or maple syrup.

Step-by-Step Instructions:

- In two bowls or glasses, arrange the yogurt or kefir, granola, and berries. Drizzle with either honey or maple syrup.
- Serve as a quick and convenient breakfast or snack.

Chia Seed Pudding with Coconut Milk and Mango

- *Servings: Two.*
- *Prep time: 5 minutes, plus overnight.*

Ingredients:

- 1/4 cup of chia seeds.
- One cup canned coconut milk.
- Two tablespoons of honey or maple syrup.
- 1/4 teaspoon of vanilla extract.
- 1/4 teaspoon of cardamom (optional)
- 1/2 cup chopped fresh or frozen mango.

Step-by-Step Instructions:

- In a small mixing bowl, combine the chia seeds, coconut milk, honey or maple syrup, vanilla, and cardamom, if desired.
- Divide the mixture into two lidded jars or containers. Top with mango. Refrigerate the lids for at least 4 hours, preferably overnight.
- Enjoy chilled or at room temperature.

<u>*Tofu Scramble with Vegetables*</u>

- ***Servings: Two.***
- ***Prep time: 15 minutes.***

Ingredients:

- One tablespoon of olive oil.
- 1/4 cup chopped onion.
- 1/4 cup diced red bell pepper.
- 1/4 cup chopped mushrooms.
- Add salt and pepper to taste.
- One-quarter teaspoon turmeric
- One-quarter teaspoon cumin
- 1/4 teaspoon of smoked paprika.
- One-quarter teaspoon garlic powder
- 8 ounces firm tofu, drained and crumbled
- Two cups baby spinach.
- Two tablespoons of nutritional yeast (optional).
- 2 pieces of whole wheat bread toasted (optional)

Step-by-Step Instructions:

- Heat oil in a large skillet over medium-high heat. Cook, stirring occasionally, until the veggies are tender, about 10 minutes.
- Stir in the turmeric, cumin, smoked paprika, and garlic powder to evenly cover the vegetables. Cook, stirring, until the spinach is wilted and the tofu is well cooked, about 5 minutes. Sprinkle with nutritional yeast if desired.
- You may serve the tofu scramble with toast or on its own.

Breakfast Burrito Bowl

- *Servings: Two.*
- *Prep time: 20 minutes.*

Ingredients:

- One cup cooked brown rice or quinoa.
- 1/4 cup salsa of your preference
- One tablespoon of olive oil.
- Four eggs, beaten
- Add salt and pepper to taste.
- 1/4 cup washed and drained black beans.

- 1/4 cup of shredded cheese (optional).
- 1/4 cup chopped avocado.
- 2 tablespoons of chopped cilantro.

Step-by-Step Instructions:

- Cook the rice or quinoa and salsa in a small saucepan over low heat, stirring regularly, until heated through.
- Heat the oil in a medium skillet over medium high heat. Stir in the eggs, salt, and pepper and simmer for about 5 minutes, or until scrambled.
- Divide the rice or quinoa mixture between two bowls and top with eggs, black beans, cheese, avocado, and cilantro. Enjoy with a fork or tortilla.

CHAPTER 4

Lunch Time Delights

Mediterranean Chickpea Salad Sandwich.

- _Serves: 4_
- _Prep time: 15 minutes._

Ingredients:

- 1/4 cup plain yogurt, or kefir
- 2 teaspoons of lemon juice.
- Two teaspoons of dried oregano.
- Add salt and pepper to taste.
- 1/4 cup of chopped fresh parsley.
- Drain and rinse 2 cups of cooked or canned chickpeas.
- 1/4 cup diced red onion.
- 1/4 cup chopped cucumber.
- 1/4 cup crumbled feta cheese.
- Eight pieces of whole wheat bread
- Four lettuce leaves.

Step-by-Step Instructions:

- In a small bowl, combine the yogurt or kefir, lemon juice, oregano, salt, and pepper. Mix in the parsley and put aside.
- In a large mixing bowl, mash the chickpeas using a fork or potato masher, leaving some pieces to add texture. Toss in the onion, cucumber, and feta cheese until combined.
- Spread the yogurt dressing evenly on four slices of bread. Top with chickpea salad and lettuce leaves. Cover with the remaining bread slices and cut into halves.
- Enjoy your sandwiches or wrap them in foil and chill until ready to eat.

Salmon and Roasted Vegetables

- *Serves: 4*
- *Prep time: 30 minutes.*

Ingredients:

- 4 salmon fillets, approximately 6 ounces each.
- Two teaspoons of olive oil.
- Add salt and pepper to taste.

- Cut 4 cups of assorted veggies into bite-sized pieces, including broccoli, cauliflower, carrots, and zucchini.
- Two teaspoons of balsamic vinegar.
- Two teaspoons of honey or maple syrup.
- Two teaspoons of dried rosemary.
- Two teaspoons of minced garlic.

Step-by-Step Instructions:

- Preheat the oven to 200°C (180°C fan) and prepare a baking sheet with parchment paper. Place the salmon fillets on the prepared baking sheet and drizzle with 1 tablespoon olive oil.
- Season with salt and pepper and bake for 15 to 20 minutes, or until the salmon is flaky and fully cooked.
- In a large mixing bowl, combine the veggies with the remaining olive oil, balsamic vinegar, honey or maple syrup, rosemary, garlic, salt, and pepper.
- Place the vegetables in a single layer on another baking sheet and roast for 15 to 20 minutes, or until soft and caramelized.
- Serve the fish beside the roasted vegetables and enjoy.

Lentil Soup and Whole-Wheat Bread

- *Serves: 4*
- *Prep time: 40 minutes.*

Ingredients:

- Two teaspoons of olive oil.
- 1 onion, chopped
- two carrots, peeled and chopped
- Two celery stalks, diced
- 2 garlic cloves, minced
- Add salt and pepper to taste.
- One teaspoon dried thyme.
- One teaspoon of dried rosemary
- Four cups of veggie broth.
- Two glasses of water.
- One 15-ounce can have diced tomatoes.
- 1 1/2 cups brown or green lentils, rinsed and drained
- Two bay leaves.
- 2 teaspoons of lemon juice.
- 4 pieces of whole wheat bread toasted (optional)

Step-by-Step Instructions:

- Warm the oil in a big pot over medium-high heat. Cook the onion, carrots, celery, garlic, salt, and pepper for about 15 minutes, stirring occasionally.
- Boil the thyme, rosemary, broth, water, tomatoes, lentils, and bay leaves. Simmer, uncovered, until the lentils are cooked, about 20 to 25 minutes.
- Discard the bay leaves and add the lemon juice. If needed, season with additional salt and pepper.
- Serve the soup with bread if desired, or eat it on its own.

Quinoa Salad with Grilled Chicken

- *Serves: 4*
- *Prep time: 30 minutes.*

Ingredients:

- 1/4 cup plain yogurt, or kefir
- 2 teaspoons of lemon juice.
- Two teaspoons of honey or maple syrup.
- Add salt and pepper to taste.
- Cut 1 pound of boneless, skinless chicken breasts into 1-inch chunks.

- Eight wooden or metal skewers.

- Two cups cooked quinoa.

- Two cups baby spinach.

- 1/4 cup of chopped fresh mint.

- 1/4 cup of chopped fresh parsley.

- 1/4 cup crumbled feta cheese.

- Two teaspoons of olive oil.

- 2 teaspoons of lemon juice.

- Add salt and pepper to taste.

Step-by-Step Instructions:

- In a small mixing bowl, combine the yogurt or kefir, lemon juice, honey or maple syrup, salt, and pepper. Set aside 2 tablespoons of the dressing for later use, and transfer the remaining to a big Ziplock bag.

- Place the chicken pieces in the bag and seal it. Refrigerate for at least 15 minutes, or up to 2 hours, rotating the bag occasionally to ensure the chicken is evenly coated.

- Preheat the grill to medium-high heat, then lightly oil the grates. Thread the chicken onto the skewers, discarding the marinade.

- Grill the skewers for 10-15 minutes, flipping occasionally, until the chicken is well roasted and blackened.
- In a large mixing bowl, combine the quinoa, spinach, mint, parsley, feta cheese, olive oil, lemon juice, salt, and pepper.
- Divide the salad among four plates and top with chicken skewers. Drizzle with the remaining dressing and enjoy.

Tuna Salad, Lettuce Wraps

- *Serves: 4*
- *Prep time: 15 minutes.*

Ingredients:

- Two 5-ounce cans of tuna, drained and flakes
- 1/4 cup plain yogurt, or kefir
- Two tablespoons of mayonnaise.
- Two teaspoons of Dijon mustard.
- Two teaspoons of lemon juice.
- Add salt and pepper to taste.
- 1/4 cup chopped celery.
- 2 tablespoons chopped fresh dill.

- 8 large lettuce leaves (romaine or butterhead)
- 1/4 cup chopped almonds (optional).

Step-by-Step Instructions:

- In a medium bowl, combine the tuna, yogurt or kefir, mayonnaise, mustard, lemon juice, salt, and pepper. Fold in the celery and dill.
- Divide the tuna salad evenly among the lettuce leaves, and top with almonds if preferred. Roll up the lettuce leaves and secure using toothpicks as needed.
- Eat your lettuce wraps immediately or store them in the refrigerator until ready to eat.

Black Bean Burgers

- *Serves: 4*
- *Prep time: 25 minutes.*

Ingredients:

- One 15-ounce can of black beans, drained and rinsed
- 1/4 cup rolled oats.
- One-quarter cup chopped onion
- 2 garlic cloves, minced
- One teaspoon cumin.

- 1/2 teaspoons smoked paprika.
- 1/4 teaspoon of salt.
- 1/4 teaspoon of black pepper.
- Two teaspoons of olive oil.
- Four whole wheat hamburger buns.
- Four lettuce leaves.
- Four tomato slices.
- Four tablespoons of salsa or ketchup.

Step-by-Step Instructions:

- In a food processor, add the black beans, oats, onion, garlic, cumin, smoked paprika, salt, and pepper. Process until well incorporated but still chunky.
- Shape the mixture into four patties and chill for 15 minutes to harden.
- Heat oil in a large skillet over medium-high heat. Cook the patties for 4 to 5 minutes on each side, or until brown and crispy.
- Serve the burgers on buns with lettuce, tomato, and salsa or ketchup. Enjoy with your favourite sides.

Chicken And Vegetable Skewers in A Yogurt Marinade.

- _Serves: 4_
- _Prep time: 30 minutes, plus marinating time._

Ingredients:

- 1/4 cup plain yogurt, or kefir
- 2 teaspoons of lemon juice.
- Two teaspoons of dried oregano.
- Two teaspoons of minced garlic.
- Add salt and pepper to taste.
- Cut 1 pound of boneless, skinless chicken breasts into 1-inch chunks.
- Two cups of cherry tomatoes.
- 2 cups zucchini, cut into half-inch rounds
- Two teaspoons of olive oil.
- Fresh parsley for garnish (optional).

Step-by-Step Instructions:

- In a small bowl, combine the yogurt or kefir, lemon juice, oregano, garlic, salt, and pepper. Set aside 2 tablespoons of the marinade for later use and transfer the remainder to a large Ziplock bag.

- Place the chicken pieces in the bag and seal it. Refrigerate for at least 2 hours, or up to overnight, rotating the bag occasionally to ensure that the chicken is evenly coated.

- Preheat the grill to medium-high heat, then lightly oil the grates. Thread the chicken, tomatoes, and zucchini onto metal or wooden skewers, leaving enough space between each.

- Brush the skewers with olive oil and sprinkle with salt and pepper.

- Grill the skewers for 10 to 15 minutes, rotating regularly, until the chicken is fully cooked and the vegetables are browned.

- Drizzle with the leftover marinade and garnish with parsley, if preferred. Serve hot or room temperature.

Leftover Veggie Curry and Brown Rice

- *Serves: 4*
- *Prep time: 20 minutes.*

Ingredients:

- Two teaspoons of coconut oil.
- 1 onion, chopped
- Two teaspoons of curry powder.
- One teaspoon of turmeric.
- One teaspoon cumin.
- One teaspoon of salt.
- 1/4 teaspoon of cayenne pepper (optional).
- 4 cups leftover cooked vegetables, such as cauliflower, carrots, potatoes, or green beans, diced
- One 15-ounce can of coconut milk.
- Two tablespoons of tomato paste.
- 2 tablespoons of chopped cilantro.
- Four cups of cooked brown rice.

Step-by-Step Instructions:

- In a large skillet over medium-high heat, melt the coconut oil. Cook the onion, turning regularly, until tender, about 10 minutes.

- Stir in the curry powder, turmeric, cumin, salt, and cayenne pepper, if using, and simmer for 1 minute, or until aromatic.
- Bring the leftover vegetables, coconut milk, and tomato paste to a boil. Reduce the heat to a simmer, stirring regularly, for about 10 minutes, or until the sauce thickens and the veggies are thoroughly heated.
- Stir in the cilantro and serve the curry with rice. Enjoy with naan bread or yogurt, if desired.

Greek Yogurt Bowl with Berries & Granola

- *Servings: Two.*
- *Prep time: 5 minutes.*

Ingredients:

- Two cups plain yogurt or kefir.
- Two tablespoons of honey or maple syrup.
- 1/4 teaspoon of vanilla extract.
- One-quarter teaspoon cinnamon
- 1 cup fresh or frozen mixed berries.
- 1/4 cup granola of your preference

Step-by-Step Instructions:

- In a small mixing bowl, combine the yogurt or kefir, honey or maple syrup, vanilla, and cinnamon.
- Divide the yogurt mixture between two bowls, then top with berries and granola. Enjoy as a refreshing and filling lunch or snack.

Avocado Toast with Eggs and Smoked Salmon.

- *Servings: Two.*
- *Prep time: 15 minutes.*

Ingredients:

- Two pieces of whole wheat bread, toasted
- One ripe avocado, peeled and pitted
- Add salt and pepper to taste.
- Two teaspoons of butter or olive oil.
- Four eggs, beaten
- Add salt and pepper to taste.
- Two ounces of smoked salmon.
- Two teaspoons of capers (optional)
- Fresh dill for garnish (optional).

Step-by-Step Instructions:

- In a small mixing bowl, mash the avocado with a fork and season with salt and pepper.
- Spread the avocado evenly on the bread slices.
- In a medium skillet over medium-high heat, melt the butter or oil. Stir in the eggs, salt, and pepper and simmer for about 5 minutes, or until scrambled.
- Spread the eggs over the avocado toast, then top with smoked salmon, capers, and dill if desired. Enjoy with a fork and knife or by hand.

CHAPTER 5

Dinner

Sheet Pan Chicken Fajita Bowls

- *Servings: four.*
- *Prepare time: 15 minutes.*
- *Cook for 25 minutes.*

Ingredients:

- One tablespoon of chili powder.
- One teaspoon of ground cumin
- Salt and pepper to taste.
- Two tablespoons of olive or canola oil.
- 1 1/2 pounds boneless and skinless chicken breasts, sliced 1/4 inch thick.
- Cut 1 red bell pepper into 1/2-inch-thick pieces.
- Cut 1 yellow bell pepper into 1/2-inch-thick pieces.
- One large red onion, sliced 1/2 inch thick.
- One 15-ounce can have rinsed and drained black beans.
- 4 tablespoons fresh lime juice (from approximately two limes)

- 1/2 cup sour cream.

- 1/2 cup of fresh cilantro, roughly chopped

- Four cups of cooked brown rice.

Step-by-Step Instructions:

- Preheat the oven to 425°F. Line a rimmed baking sheet with foil.

- In a small bowl, combine the chili powder, cumin, salt, pepper, and oil.

- In a large mixing bowl, combine the chicken, peppers, and onion with the spice mixture.

- Spread the chicken and veggies evenly on the prepared baking sheet and bake for 15 minutes, or until the chicken is fully cooked and the vegetables are soft.

- Meanwhile, in a small saucepan over low heat, combine the black beans and 2 tablespoons lime juice, stirring occasionally.

- In a separate bowl, combine the sour cream, cilantro, and remaining 2 tablespoons lime juice. Season with salt and pepper to taste.

- To serve, divide the rice into four dishes and top with the chicken and vegetable mixture. Place some black beans in each bowl and drizzle with the sour cream sauce.

Three-Beans Chili

- *Servings: six.*
- *Prep time is 10 minutes.*
- *Cook for 45 minutes.*

Ingredients:

- 1/2 cup minced onion.
- 1/2 cup chopped green pepper.
- 1/2 cup of celery, chopped
- 1 teaspoon minced garlic.
- One tablespoon of olive oil.
- 28 oz canned crushed tomatoes.
- 14 1/2 oz canned Mexican chopped tomatoes.
- 1/4 cup chopped sun-dried tomatoes (not packed with oil)
- 15 ounces of canned pinto beans, rinsed and drained
- Rinse and drain 16 ounces of canned kidney beans.
- 15 oz canned black beans, rinsed and drained.
- 1/2 cup of dark beer.
- One tablespoon of chili powder.

- Two teaspoons of baking cocoa.
- 1 cup shredded Mexican cheese blend.

Step-by-Step Instructions:

• Heat the oil in a large pot over medium-high heat, then sauté the onion, green pepper, celery, and garlic for 10 minutes, or until crisp-tender.

• Combine tomatoes, beans, beer, chili powder, and chocolate. Bring to a boil, then reduce to a simmer, covered, for 40 minutes, stirring regularly.

• Optional: serve with cheese on top.

Spinach and Artichoke Dip Pasta

- *Servings: four.*
- *Prep time is 10 minutes.*
- *Cook for 20 minutes.*

Ingredients:

- 8 ounces of whole wheat penne pasta.
- One tablespoon of olive oil.
- One-quarter cup chopped onion
- 2 garlic cloves, minced
- 1/4 teaspoon of salt.

- 1/4 teaspoon of black pepper.

- Softened 8-ounces of reduced-fat cream cheese

- 1/4 cup of low-fat milk.

- 1/4 cup grated parmesan cheese.

- 1/4 teaspoon of dried oregano.

- One-quarter teaspoon of dried basil

- 10 oz frozen chopped spinach, thawed and pressed dry.

- 14 ounces of canned artichoke hearts, drained and chopped

Step-by-Step Instructions:

- Cook the pasta according to package instructions, then drain and return it to the saucepan.

- Heat the oil in a large skillet over medium heat. Cook the onion, garlic, salt, and pepper for about 5 minutes, or until tender.

- In a small bowl, combine the cream cheese, milk, Parmesan, oregano, and basil. Whisk until smooth.

- Combine the cream cheese mixture, spinach, and artichokes in the skillet. Cook for about 10 minutes on low heat, stirring occasionally.

- Toss the pasta in the skillet to coat with the sauce. Serve hot or room temperature.

Roasted Salmon with Smoked Chickpeas and Greens.

- *Servings: four.*
- *Prepare time: 15 minutes.*
- *Cook for 25 minutes.*

Ingredients:

- Two tablespoons of extra virgin olive oil, split
- One tablespoon of smoked paprika.
- 1/2 teaspoon salt, divided, and a pinch
- 1 (15 ounce) can washed chickpeas with no salt added.
- One-third cup buttermilk
- One-quarter cup mayonnaise
- 1/4 cup chopped fresh chives and/or dill, plus extra to garnish.
- 1/2 teaspoon of ground pepper, divided
- One-quarter teaspoon garlic powder
- 10 cups of chopped kale.
- One-quarter cup water
- 1 1/4 pounds of wild salmon, divided into four parts

Step-by-Step Instructions:

- Preheat the oven to 425°F. Line a rimmed baking sheet with foil.

- In a small bowl, combine the oil, paprika, and 1/4 teaspoon salt.

- Toss the chickpeas in a large basin with the oil mixture until thoroughly coated.

- Spread the chickpeas on the prepared baking sheet and bake on the higher rack for 30 minutes, stirring twice.

- Meanwhile, in a separate bowl, combine the buttermilk, mayonnaise, herbs, 1/4 teaspoon pepper, and garlic powder. Set aside.

- Heat the remaining 1 tablespoon oil in a large skillet over medium heat and sauté the kale for 2 minutes, turning periodically. Add the water and simmer for another 5 minutes, or until the kale is soft. Season with a pinch of salt.

- Remove the chickpeas from the oven and place them on one side of the pan. Place the salmon on the opposite side and season with the remaining 1/4 teaspoon salt and pepper.

- Bake the salmon for 5 to 8 minutes, or until just cooked through.

- Drizzle the remaining dressing over the salmon, garnish with additional herbs if preferred, and serve alongside the kale and chickpeas.

Miso Soup Cup of Noodles with Shrimp and Green Tea Soba.

- **_Servings: three._**
- **_Prepare time: 15 minutes._**
- **_Cook for 10 minutes._**

Ingredients:

- Four tablespoons of white miso.
- Six teaspoons of mirin.
- Three teaspoons of unseasoned rice vinegar.
- 1 1/2 cups diagonally cut snow peas (about 5 ounces)
- 9 ounces peeled, cooked shrimp
- 1 1/2 teaspoons of dried wakame (see Tip)
- 1 1/2 cups cooked green tea soba noodles (from 3-4 ounces dried; refer to Tip)
- Three teaspoons of thinly sliced scallions
- 1 (3-inch) square dried kombu cut into three equal strips (see Tip)
- 3 cups extremely hot water, divided

Step-by-Step Instructions:

- In three 1 1/2-pint canning jars, combine 1 tablespoon + 1 teaspoon miso, 2 teaspoons mirin, and 1 teaspoon vinegar.
- Place 1/2 cup snow peas, 3 ounces shrimp, 1/2 teaspoon wakame, and 1/2 cup noodles in each container.
- Garnish each with 1 tablespoon scallions.
- Place a piece of kombu between the ingredients and the side of each jar.
- Cover and refrigerate for up to three days.
- To prepare each jar, add 1 cup of extremely hot water, cover, and shake vigorously to dissolve the miso.
- Uncover and microwave in 1-minute increments on High until steaming hot, about 2 to 3 minutes. Discard the kombu.
- Stir to ensure that the miso has dissolved. Allow to stand for a few minutes before eating.

<u>*Vegetarian Enchiladas Casserole*</u>

- *Servings: six.*
- *Prepare time: 15 minutes.*
- *Cook for 30 minutes.*

Ingredients:

- 1/2 cup minced onion.
- 1/2 cup chopped green pepper.
- 1/2 cup of celery, chopped
- 1 teaspoon minced garlic.
- One tablespoon of olive oil.
- 28 oz canned crushed tomatoes.
- 14 1/2 oz canned Mexican chopped tomatoes.
- 1/4 cup chopped sun-dried tomatoes (not packed with oil)
- 15 ounces of canned pinto beans, rinsed and drained
- Rinse and drain 16 ounces of canned kidney beans.
- 15 oz canned black beans, rinsed and drained.
- 1/2 cup of dark beer.
- One tablespoon of chili powder.
- Two teaspoons of baking cocoa.
- 1 cup shredded Mexican cheese blend.

Step-by-Step Instructions:

- Heat the oil in a large pot over medium-high heat, then sauté the onion, green pepper, celery, and garlic for 10 minutes, or until crisp-tender.
- Combine tomatoes, beans, beer, chili powder, and chocolate. Bring to a boil, then reduce to a simmer, covered, for 20 minutes, stirring regularly.
- Preheat the oven to 375°F. Spray a 9x13 inch baking dish with cooking spray.
- Place half of the bean mixture in the prepared dish and sprinkle with half of the cheese. Repeat with the remaining beans and cheese.
- Bake for 10 minutes, or until the cheese melts and bubbles.
- Optional garnishes include sour cream, cilantro, and tortilla chips.

Hearty Chickpea and Spinach Stew

- *Servings: four.*
- *Prep time is 10 minutes.*
- *Cook for 20 minutes.*

Ingredients:

- Two tablespoons of extra virgin olive oil, split
- One tablespoon of smoked paprika.
- 1/2 teaspoon salt, divided, and a pinch
- 1 (15 ounce) can washed chickpeas with no salt added.
- One-third cup buttermilk
- One-quarter cup mayonnaise
- 1/4 cup chopped fresh chives and/or dill, plus extra to garnish.
- 1/2 teaspoon of ground pepper, divided
- One-quarter teaspoon garlic powder
- 10 cups of chopped kale.
- One-quarter cup water
- 1 1/4 pounds of wild salmon, divided into four parts

Step-by-Step Instructions:

- Preheat the oven to 425°F. Line a rimmed baking sheet with foil.

- In a small bowl, combine the oil, paprika, and 1/4 teaspoon salt.

- Toss the chickpeas in a large basin with the oil mixture until thoroughly coated.

- Spread the chickpeas on the prepared baking sheet and bake on the higher rack for 30 minutes, stirring twice.

- Meanwhile, in a separate bowl, combine the buttermilk, mayonnaise, herbs, 1/4 teaspoon pepper, and garlic powder. Set aside.

- Heat the remaining 1 tablespoon oil in a large skillet over medium heat and sauté the kale for 2 minutes, turning periodically.

- Add the water and simmer for another 5 minutes, or until the kale is soft. Season with a pinch of salt.

- Remove the chickpeas from the oven and place them on one side of the pan. Place the salmon on the opposite side and season with the remaining 1/4 teaspoon salt and pepper.

- Bake the salmon for 5 to 8 minutes, or until just cooked through.

- Drizzle the leftover dressing over the salmon, sprinkle with additional herbs if preferred, and serve alongside the greens and chickpeas.

Baked Garlic Salmon Balls

- *Servings: four.*
- *Prep time is 10 minutes.*
- *Cook for 20 minutes.*

Ingredients:

- Two (6-ounce) cans of boneless, skinless salmon, drained
- Three tablespoons of Italian breadcrumbs.
- 1 finely sliced scallion.
- One big egg, lightly beaten
- 1 tablespoon of low-fat plain strained yogurt, such Greek-style.
- 1 tablespoon of minced garlic.
- Cooking Spray

Step-by-Step Instructions:

- Preheat the oven to 400 degrees Fahrenheit and line a large rimmed baking sheet with parchment paper.

- In a large bowl, combine the salmon, breadcrumbs, scallions, egg, yogurt, and garlic; toss until well combined, breaking up the fish.

- Using clean hands, form approximately 1 1/2 tablespoons of the dough into a ball and place on the prepared baking sheet. Repeat with the remaining ingredients to make 18 to 20 salmon balls.

- Lightly spray the balls with cooking spray.

- Bake for approximately 20 minutes, flipping once, until firm and brown.

- Serve with lemon wedges, salad, or your preferred sauce.

Beetroot Hummus

- ***Serves: 8***
- ***Prepare time: 15 minutes.***

Ingredients:

- One teaspoon of cumin seeds.

- 250g (9 oz) cooked beetroot, drained and quartered

- 400g canned chickpeas, drained and rinsed.

- One garlic clove, peeled

- One teaspoon of ground coriander.

- 1/2 teaspoon flaky sea salt, to taste.

- Two teaspoons of extra virgin olive oil.

- 2 teaspoons of fresh lemon juice.

- Ground black pepper.

Step-by-Step Instructions:

- Gently toast the cumin seeds in a small dry frying pan for 2 minutes, stirring periodically, before removing from heat.

- Place the beetroot, chickpeas, garlic, coriander, salt, and olive oil in a food processor. Add the cumin seeds and lemon juice, and season with freshly ground black pepper.

- Blitz until smooth. Check the seasoning to taste, adding more salt, pepper, or lemon juice as needed, and blitz again.

- Serve the hummus as a spread on sandwiches and wraps, or as dip. Store covered in the refrigerator for up to three days, or freeze.

Vegan Pasta Bake

- *Servings: six*
- *Prepare time: 15 minutes*
- *Cook for 25 minutes*

Ingredients:

- 12 ounces of whole wheat penne pasta.
- One tablespoon of olive oil.
- 1 onion, diced
- 2 garlic cloves, minced
- 1/4 teaspoon red pepper flakes (optional)
- Two cups marinara sauce.
- 1/4 cup nutritional yeast.
- 2 tablespoons fresh basil, chopped, plus extra for garnish.
- Salt and pepper to taste.
- Two cups baby spinach.
- 1 1/2 cups shredded vegan mozzarella.

Step-by-Step Instructions:

- Preheat the oven to 375°F. Spray a 9x13 inch baking dish with cooking spray.
- Cook the pasta according to package instructions, then drain and return it to the saucepan.

- Heat the oil in a large skillet over medium-high heat, then cook the onion, garlic, and red pepper flakes (if using) until soft, about 10 minutes.

- Boil the marinara sauce, nutritional yeast, basil, salt, and pepper. Reduce the heat to a simmer for 5 minutes, stirring occasionally.

- Add the spinach and cook for 2 minutes, or until wilted.

- Toss the pasta with the sauce until well combined. Transfer the pasta mixture to the prepared baking dish and top with the vegan cheese.

- Bake for 15 minutes, or until the cheese melts and bubbles.

- If desired, garnish with extra basil and serve hot or at room temperature.

CHAPTER 6

Snacks

Carrot and Banana Muffins

- *Serves: 16*
- *Prep time: 15 minutes.*

Ingredients:

- Two cups all-purpose flour.
- 1/4 cup granulated sugar.
- One-quarter cup brown sugar
- Two teaspoons of baking powder.
- One teaspoon of cinnamon.
- 1/4 teaspoon of salt.
- 1/4 cup unsalted butter melted
- Two eggs, lightly beaten
- One teaspoon of vanilla extract.
- 1 1/2 cups shredded carrots.
- Two ripe bananas, mashed
- 1/4 cup of chopped pecans (optional)

Step-by-Step Instructions:

- Preheat the oven to 375°F. Line a 12-cup muffin tray with paper liners. In a large basin, combine the flour, sugars, baking powder, cinnamon, and salt.

- In a medium bowl, combine the butter, eggs, vanilla, carrots, and bananas.

- Mix the wet ingredients into the dry ingredients until just mixed. Fold in the pecans, if using.

- Divide the batter evenly among the prepared muffin cups, filling each about 3/4 full.

- Bake for 18–20 minutes, or until a toothpick inserted in the centre comes out clean.

- Let the muffins cool in the pan for 10 minutes before transferring to a wire rack to cool fully. For an added boost of protein, pair with some yogurt or peanut butter.

<u>*Crunchy Roasted Chickpeas*</u>

- *Serves: 4*
- *Prep time: 5 minutes.*

Ingredients:

- One (15-ounce) can of chickpeas, drained and rinsed
- One tablespoon of olive oil.
- 1/2 teaspoon of salt.
- 1/4 teaspoon paprika.
- One-quarter teaspoon garlic powder
- One-quarter teaspoon cumin
- 1/8 teaspoon of cayenne pepper (optional).

Step-by-Step Instructions:

- Preheat the oven to 400°F. Line a baking sheet with parchment paper.
- Pat the chickpeas dry with paper towels before spreading them in a single layer on the prepared baking sheet.
- Drizzle olive oil over chickpeas and toss to coat. Season with salt, paprika, garlic powder, cumin, and cayenne pepper, if using. Toss again to evenly distribute the spices.

- Bake for 25–30 minutes, stirring once or twice, until the chickpeas are golden and crispy.
- Allow them to cool somewhat before eating as a snack or salad topping.

Black Bean Hummus

- *Servings: eight.*
- *Prep time: 10 minutes.*

Ingredients:

- One (15-ounce) can of black beans, drained and rinsed
- 1/4 cup tahini.
- One-quarter cup lemon juice
- Two teaspoons of olive oil.
- 2 garlic cloves, peeled
- 1/2 teaspoon of salt.
- One-quarter teaspoon cumin
- 1/4 teaspoon paprika.
- 2 teaspoons of minced fresh cilantro (optional).

Step-by-Step Instructions:

- Combine the black beans, tahini, lemon juice, olive oil, garlic, salt, cumin, and paprika in a food processor; process until smooth and creamy, scraping down the sides as needed.
- If the hummus is too thick for you, thin it out with water.
- Place the hummus in a serving bowl and sprinkle with cilantro if desired. Serve alongside fresh vegetables, whole wheat pita bread, or tortilla chips.

Apple Wedges with Peanut Butter

- *Servings: Two.*
- *Prep time: 5 minutes.*

Ingredients:

- One large apple, cored and cut into sixteen wedges.
- Two tablespoons of natural peanut butter.
- 1/4 teaspoon of ground cinnamon (optional).
- Step-by-Step Instructions:
  - Place the apple wedges on a big plate or platter. Sprinkle with cinnamon if desired.

- Place the peanut butter in a small microwave-safe bowl and heat for 10 to 15 seconds, or until slightly melted and smooth.
- Drizzle the peanut butter over the apple wedges or use as a dip on the side. Enjoy this crunchy and creamy snack high in fibre and protein.

Strawberry Fruit Salad.

- *Serves: 4*
- *Prep time: 15 minutes.*

Ingredients:

- 2 cups freshly hulled and halved strawberries.
- One cup of fresh blueberries
- One cup of fresh pineapple pieces
- 1/4 cup fresh mint leaves, chopped
- Two teaspoons of honey.
- 2 teaspoons of lemon juice.

Step-by-Step Instructions:

- In a large bowl, combine the strawberries, blueberries, pineapple, and mint.

- In a small bowl, mix together the honey and lemon juice until thoroughly incorporated.

- Pour the honey-lemon dressing over the fruit salad and gently toss to coat. Refrigerate until ready to serve or eat straight away.

- This vibrant and refreshing salad is rich in vitamin C and antioxidants.

Tropical Fruit and Nut Snack

- *Serves: 4*
- *Prep time: 10 minutes.*

Ingredients:

- 1/4 cup unsalted cashews.
- 1/4 cup unsalted macadamia nuts.
- 1/4 cup unsweetened, shredded coconut
- 1/4 cup dried mango, chopped
- 1/4 cup dried pineapple, chopped
- 1/4 cup of dried banana chips.

Step-by-Step Instructions:

- Toast the cashews, macadamia nuts, and coconut in a small skillet over medium-low heat for 5 to 7 minutes, or until brown and aromatic.
- Stir often. Transfer to a large bowl and allow it cool somewhat.
- Toss in the dried mango, pineapple, and banana chips. Keep in an airtight jar at room temperature for up to a week.
- Enjoy this tropical snack mix, which is crispy, chewy, and delightful.

Guacamole and Dippers

- *Serves: 4*
- *Prep time: 10 minutes.*

Ingredients:

- Two ripe avocados, peeled and pitted.
- 1/4 cup diced red onion
- 1/4 cup of chopped fresh cilantro.
- Two teaspoons of lime juice.
- 1/2 teaspoon of salt.
- One-quarter teaspoon cumin

- One-quarter teaspoon garlic powder

- 1/8 teaspoon of black pepper.

- Dippers of your choice: carrot sticks, celery sticks, cucumber slices, bell pepper strips, whole wheat crackers, or baked tortilla chips.

Step-by-Step Instructions:

- In a medium bowl, mash the avocados with a fork until they are somewhat chunky.

- Combine the onion, cilantro, lime juice, salt, cumin, garlic powder, and black pepper. Taste and adjust seasoning as needed.

- Place the guacamole in a serving basin and serve with your favourite dippers.

- Enjoy this creamy, delicious snack high in healthy fats and fibre.

Homemade Trail Mix

- *Servings: eight.*
- *Prep time: 5 minutes.*

Ingredients:

- One-quarter cup raw almonds
- One-quarter cup raw walnuts
- 1/4 cup uncooked pumpkin seeds
- 1/4 cup dried cranberries.
- 1/4 cup of dark chocolate chips.

Step-by-Step Instructions:

- In a large bowl, combine the almonds, walnuts, pumpkin seeds, cranberries, and chocolate chips.
- Keep in an airtight jar at room temperature for up to a week.
- Enjoy this crunchy, sweet snack high in protein and antioxidants.

Toasted Paprika Chickpeas

- *Serves: 4*
- *Prep time: 5 minutes.*

Ingredients:

- One (15-ounce) can of chickpeas, drained and rinsed
- One tablespoon of olive oil.
- 1/2 teaspoon of salt.
- 1/4 teaspoon paprika.
- One-quarter teaspoon garlic powder
- One-quarter teaspoon cumin
- 1/8 teaspoon of cayenne pepper (optional).

Step-by-Step Instructions:

- Preheat the oven to 400°F. Line a baking sheet with parchment paper. Pat the chickpeas dry with paper towels before spreading them in a single layer on the prepared baking sheet.
- Drizzle olive oil over chickpeas and toss to coat. Season with salt, paprika, garlic powder, cumin, and cayenne pepper, if using. Toss again to evenly distribute the spices.
- Bake for 25–30 minutes, stirring once or twice, until the chickpeas are golden and crispy.

- Allow them to cool slightly before eating as a snack or salad topping.

Air-Fried Cinnamon-Ginger Apple Chips

- *Serves: 4*
- *Prep time: 10 minutes.*

Ingredients:

- Two large apples, cored and thinly sliced
- 1/4 teaspoon of ground cinnamon.
- 1/4 teaspoon of ground ginger.
- Cooking Spray

Step-by-Step Instructions:

- Preheat an air fryer to 300 degrees Fahrenheit and coat the basket with cooking spray.
- Arrange the apple slices in a single layer in the basket, working in batches as needed. Sprinkle with cinnamon and ginger.
- Air-fry the apple slices for 15 to 20 minutes, flipping halfway through, until crispy and golden. Transfer to a wire rack and cool fully.
- Enjoy these crunchy and spicy apple chips, which are low in calories yet high in taste.

CHAPTER 7

Desserts

Kefir, Banana, Almond, And Frozen Berry Smoothie.

- *Servings: Two.*
- *Prep time: 5 minutes.*

Ingredients:

- One ripe banana.
- 350 mL kefir.
- 75 g frozen mixed berries.
- 40 grams whole almonds
- One tablespoon maple syrup or runny honey.

Step-by-Step Instructions:

- Place everything in a blender or food processor and process until perfectly smooth.
- Pour into two glasses and serve.

Strawberry-Mango Nice Cream.

- *Serves: 4*
- *Prep time: 10 minutes.*

Ingredients:

- 12 oz frozen mango pieces.
- 8 ounces of frozen sliced strawberries.
- One tablespoon of lime juice.

Step-by-Step Instructions:

- Combine mango, strawberries, and lime juice in a food processor; process for 1 to 2 minutes. Stop the processor and scrape the sides.
- Process for an additional 2 to 3 minutes until smooth, adding up to 1/2 cup water as needed to help process the fruit.
- Transfer to a freezer-safe container and freeze until hard, or serve as soft-serve.

Quick Strawberry Cheesecake

- *Servings: eight.*
- *Prep time: 15 minutes.*

Ingredients:

- 1 1/4 cup Graham cracker crumbs
- 1/3 cup melted butter.
- One-quarter cup white sugar
- Two teaspoons of ground cinnamon.
- Two (10-ounce) packets of frozen sweetened sliced strawberries, thawed and drained
- Two teaspoons of cornstarch.
- Two (8-ounce) packets of softened cream cheese
- One (14-ounce) can of sweetened condensed milk
- One-quarter cup lemon juice
- One teaspoon of vanilla extract.
- 2 eggs

Step-by-Step Instructions:

- Preheat the oven to 350°F. In a small bowl, combine the graham cracker crumbs, butter, sugar, and cinnamon.

- Press onto the bottom and sides of a 9-inch springform pan. Bake for 8 minutes, then cool slightly.

- In a blender or food processor, combine the strawberries and cornstarch until smooth. Transfer to a small saucepan and bring to a boil over medium-high heat while stirring frequently.

- Cook for approximately 2 minutes, or until thickened. Allow to cool slightly.

- In a large mixing bowl, use an electric mixer to beat the cream cheese until smooth. Gradually add the condensed milk, lemon juice, and vanilla.

- Add the eggs one at a time, beating thoroughly after each addition.

- Pour half of the cream cheese mixture onto the crust. Spread half of the strawberry sauce over the cream cheese layer.

- Carefully distribute the remaining cream cheese mixture over the strawberry layer. Drop spoonful of the leftover strawberry sauce on top and swirl with a knife.

- Bake for 25-30 minutes, or until the middle is nearly set. Cool on a wire rack and chill for at least 4 hours before serving.

Bev's Chocolate Chip Cookies

- *Serves: 30.*
- *Prep time: 15 minutes.*

Ingredients:

- 3/4 cup rolled oats.
- One cup of whole wheat flour.
- 1/2 teaspoon of baking soda.
- 1/2 teaspoon of salt.
- 1/4 cup softened butter.
- One-quarter cup canola oil
- 1/3 cup granulated sugar.
- One-third cup brown sugar
- One big egg.
- One teaspoon of vanilla extract.
- One cup of chocolate chips.

Step-by-Step Instructions:

- Preheat the oven to 350°F. Coat two baking sheets with cooking spray.
- Grind the oats in a blender or food processor. Transfer to a medium bowl and mix in the flour, baking soda, and salt.

- In a large mixing basin, use an electric mixer to beat the butter until creamy. Combine the oil, granulated sugar, brown sugar, egg, and vanilla; beat until smooth and creamy.

- With the mixer running, add the dry ingredients and beat on low until barely mixed. Stir in the chocolate chips.

- Drop heaping teaspoonfuls of dough onto the prepared baking sheets, leaving at least an inch between each.

- Bake the cookies, one sheet at a time, until firm around the edges and golden on top, about 15 minutes.

- Cool the cookies for 2 minutes on the baking sheets before transferring them to wire racks to cool completely.

Frozen Chocolate Coconut Milk with Strawberries

- *Serves: 4*
- *Prep time: 10 minutes.*

Ingredients:

- Two cups of frozen strawberries.
- 1 (13.5 ounce) can of coconut milk.
- Two tablespoons of honey or maple syrup.

Step-by-Step Instructions:

- Blend the frozen strawberries, coconut milk, and honey until smooth. Taste and apply extra sweetener if desired.
- Transfer the mixture to a freezer-safe container (I used a loaf pan covered with plastic wrap and foil), seal tightly, and freeze for at least 3 hours.
- Indulge in this creamy and delicious dairy-free and vegan dessert.

Red Wine Ice Cream Float.

- *Serves: 4*
- *Prep time: 5 minutes.*

Ingredients:

- Four cups of vanilla ice cream.
- 20 oz red wine.
- One cup of club soda or seltzer.
- 16 fresh, sliced strawberries

Step-by-Step Instructions:

- Scoop ice cream into four large wine glasses or mugs.
- Pour approximately 5 ounces of red wine into each glass, allowing some room at the top.
- Pour 1/4 cup club soda or seltzer into each glass and gently swirl to make some froth.
- Garnish with sliced strawberries and serve this festive dessert for Valentine's Day, Mother's Day, or any special event.

CHAPTER 8

Two-Week Meal Plan

Week 1

Monday

- Breakfast: Berry Chia Seed Overnight Oatmeal.
- Lunch: Mediterranean Chickpea Salad Sandwich.
- Dinner is Sheet-Pan Chicken Fajita Bowls.
- Snack: Carrot and banana muffins.
- Dessert: A kefir, banana, almond, and frozen fruit smoothie.

Tuesday

- Breakfast: Scrambled eggs, spinach, and tomatoes.
- Lunch: Salmon and Roasted Vegetables
- Dinner: Three-bean chili.
- Snack: crunchy roasted chickpeas.
- Dessert: Strawberry-Mango Nice Cream.

Wednesday

- Breakfast: Green smoothie bowl.
- Lunch: Lentil Soup and Whole Wheat Bread.
- Dinner: Spinach and Artichoke Dip Pasta.
- Snack: Black bean hummus.

- Dessert: quick strawberry cheesecake

Thursday

- Breakfast: baked sweet potatoes with nut butter and sliced apples.
- Lunch: Quinoa salad with grilled chicken.
- Dinner: Roasted salmon with smoked chickpeas and greens.
- Snack: Apple wedges with peanut butter.
- Dessert is Dark Chocolate Hummus.

Friday

- Breakfast: Quinoa porridge with berries and nuts.
- Lunch: Tuna salad lettuce wraps.
- Dinner: Miso Soup Cup Noodles with Shrimp and Green Tea Soba.
- Snack: Strawberry fruit salad.
- Dessert: Lemon-blueberry dump cake.

Saturday

- Breakfast: Avocado toast with sprouts and smoked salmon.
- Lunch: Black Bean Burgers.
- Dinner: vegetarian enchilada casserole.
- Snack: Tropical Fruits and Nuts.

- Dessert: Cinnamon Icebox Cookies.

Sunday

- Breakfast: Yogurt parfait with granola and fruit.
- Lunch: Chicken and vegetable skewers with yogurt marinade
- Dinner: A hearty chickpea and spinach stew.
- Snack: Guacamole and Dippers.
- Dessert: Bev's Chocolate Chip Cookies.

Week 2

Monday

- Breakfast: Chia seed pudding with coconut milk and mango.
- Lunch: Leftover Veggie Curry and Brown Rice
- Dinner: Baked Garlic Salmon Balls.
- Snack: homemade trail mix.
- Dessert: Frozen chocolate-coconut milk with strawberries.

Tuesday

- Breakfast: Tofu scramble with vegetables
- Lunch: Greek yogurt bowl with berries and granola.

- Dinner: Beetroot Hummus.
- Snack: toasted paprika chickpeas.
- Dessert: Red Wine Ice Cream Float.

Wednesday

- Breakfast: Burrito Bowl
- Lunch: Avocado toast with eggs and smoked salmon.
- Dinner: Vegan Pasta Bake.
- Snack: Air-Fried Cinnamon-Ginger Apple Chips.
- Dessert: Mug brownie.

Thursday

- Breakfast: Berry Chia Seed Overnight Oatmeal.
- Lunch: Mediterranean Chickpea Salad Sandwich.
- Dinner is Sheet-Pan Chicken Fajita Bowls.
- Snack: Carrot and banana muffins.
- Dessert: A kefir, banana, almond, and frozen fruit smoothie.

Friday

- Breakfast: Scrambled eggs, spinach, and tomatoes.
- Lunch: Salmon and Roasted Vegetables
- Dinner: Three-bean chili.
- Snack: crunchy roasted chickpeas.
- Dessert: Strawberry-Mango Nice Cream.

Saturday

- Breakfast: Green smoothie bowl.
- Lunch: Lentil Soup and Whole Wheat Bread.
- Dinner: Spinach and Artichoke Dip Pasta.
- Snack: Black bean hummus.
- Dessert: quick strawberry cheesecake

Sunday

- Breakfast: baked sweet potatoes with nut butter and sliced apples.
- Lunch: Quinoa salad with grilled chicken.
- Dinner: Roasted salmon with smoked chickpeas and greens.
- Snack: Apple wedges with peanut butter.
- Dessert is Dark Chocolate Hummus.

Exercise and Gut Health

Exercise benefits not only your muscles, heart, and lungs, but also your gut. According to research, frequent physical activity can boost the diversity and function of your gut microbiome, a community of billions of microorganisms that live in your digestive tract.

These microorganisms have critical roles in digestion, immunity, metabolism, and mood, and can be altered by a variety of factors including diet, stress, medicine, and heredity.

Exercise can help change your gut microbiota in positive ways by encouraging the growth of beneficial bacteria, lowering inflammation, increasing gut barrier function, and altering the gut-brain axis.

Here are a few ways that exercise can help your gut health:

• **Exercise can boost the variety and number of good bacteria in your gut**. A diversified and healthy gut microbiota is linked to improved health outcomes, including a lower risk of obesity, diabetes, cardiovascular disease, and inflammatory bowel disease.

Exercise can assist to populate the gut microbiome with bacteria that produce short-chain fatty acids (SCFAs), including butyrate, propionate, and acetate. SCFAs are the primary energy source for the cells that line the colon and have anti-inflammatory, anti-cancer, and anti-obesity properties.

Exercise can also boost the production of microorganisms that create other beneficial metabolites including bile acids, indole, and tryptophan, which can influence cholesterol metabolism, hormone regulation, and neurotransmitter synthesis.

Exercise can also reduce the number of bacteria that produce toxic compounds like lipopolysaccharides (LPS), which can cause inflammation and damage gut barrier function.

• **Exercise can help reduce inflammation in the intestines and throughout the body**. Inflammation is a natural immune response to injury or infection, but persistent or severe inflammation can harm the gut lining, disturb the gut flora, and contribute to a variety of disorders, including inflammatory bowel disease, irritable bowel syndrome, obesity, diabetes, and depression.

Exercise can help reduce inflammation by regulating the immune system, lowering oxidative stress, and increasing the production of anti-inflammatory cytokines like interleukin-10 (IL-10). Exercise can also lower pro-inflammatory cytokines including TNF-alpha, IL-6, and IL-1 beta, which can affect gut barrier function and change the gut flora.

• **Exercise can enhance gut barrier function and integrity**. The gut barrier is a layer of cells and mucus that separates the gut lumen from the surrounding tissues and blood vessels. It works as a selective filter, allowing nutrients and water to flow through while keeping bacteria, poisons, and allergens out.

A robust gut barrier is critical for regulating gut homeostasis and preventing systemic inflammation and illness. Exercise can help reinforce the gut barrier by raising the production of tight junction proteins like occludin and claudin, which close the gaps between gut epithelial cells.

Exercise can also stimulate the production of mucus and secretory immunoglobulin A (sIgA), which form a protective layer on the gut's surface and neutralize dangerous compounds. Exercise can also increase blood flow and oxygen delivery to the gut, improving the function and survival of gut epithelial cells.

• **Exercise can affect the gut-brain axis**. The gut-brain axis is a bidirectional communication system that connects the gut and the central nervous system via neuronal, hormonal, and immunological pathways.

The gut microbiome is an important component of the gut-brain axis because it produces neurotransmitters like serotonin, dopamine, and gamma-aminobutyric acid (GABA), which influence mood, cognition, and behaviour.

Exercise can affect the gut-brain axis by modifying gut microbiota composition and function, as well as stimulating the vagus nerve, the primary neurological channel that connects the gut and the brain. Exercise can also boost levels of brain-derived neurotrophic factor (BDNF), a protein that promotes neuronal and synaptic development and survival.

Exercise can help reduce cortisol levels, a stress hormone that can disrupt the gut-brain axis. Exercise can so benefit people's mental health and well-being by lowering stress, anxiety, and depression while also improving memory, learning, and neuroplasticity.

To summarize, exercise can benefit your gut health by increasing the diversity and function of your gut microbiome, lowering inflammation, improving gut barrier function, and altering the gut-brain axis. These advantages can lead to improved physical and mental health outcomes, such as a reduced risk of obesity, diabetes, cardiovascular disease, inflammatory bowel disease, irritable bowel syndrome, and depression.

To reap the benefits of exercise for your gut health, it is recommended that you engage in moderate to strenuous cardiovascular exercise for at least 150 minutes each week, or 30 minutes per day, five days a week.

You can also incorporate some resistance or strength training, such as lifting weights, doing push-ups, or using resistance bands, on at least two days per week.

You should also change your training program to engage different muscle groups and prevent boredom. You should also contact with your doctor before beginning any new fitness routine, especially if you have any medical concerns or injuries.

Finally, you should supplement your activity with healthy and balanced diet rich in fibre, fruits, vegetables, whole grains, legumes, nuts, seeds, and fermented foods like yogurt, kefir, sauerkraut, kimchi, and kombucha, which can help with gut health and overall well-being.

CONCLUSION

You've finished this book, but hopefully it's not the end of your road to better gut health. You should have learnt about the importance of your gut microbiome, the variables that influence it, and the foods and habits that can help it thrive. You should also have tried several delicious and simple meals that are intended to improve your gut health and overall well-being.

However, this work is not intended to be read only once. It is intended to be a guide and resource that you may refer to repeatedly while you make the adjustments that will improve your life. I recommend that you embrace a gut health diet for women as a lifestyle, not a quick fix.

A healthy stomach provides physical, mental, and emotional advantages. When your stomach aligns with your body and mind, you will feel more energized, balanced, and happy.

Of course, each woman is unique, so what works for one may not work for another. That is why you should see your doctor before beginning any new diet or fitness program, especially if you have any medical issues or sensitivities.

Your doctor can help you customize your gut health plan, track your progress, and handle any difficulties that occur along the road.

I hope this book has motivated you to take control of your gut health and realize the incredible possibilities of your internal ecology. I would love to hear from you and learn more about your experience with the gut health diet for women.

Please provide favourable reviews on the book's website. Your suggestions will help me enhance the book and reach more women who can benefit from it.

Thank you for reading the book and accompanying me on this trip. I wish you the best for your gut health and beyond. Remember: a happy gut is a happy you!